Green Smoothies: The 50 Best Green Smoothie Recipes for Weight Loss

How to Make the Best Green Smoothies to Drop Pounds

Daisy Williams

This book is dedicated to my family who support me no matter what creative project I decide to do. I am inspired and blessed because of their unconditional love.

Copyright © 2014 by Speedy Publishing LLC

All rights reserved. No part of this publication may be reproduced, distributed or transmitted in any form or by any means, including photocopying, recording, or other electronic or mechanical methods, without the prior written permission of the publisher, except in the case of brief quotations embodied in critical reviews and certain other noncommercial uses permitted by copyright law. For permission requests, write to the publisher, addressed "Attention: Permissions Coordinator," at the address below.

Speedy Publishing LLC (c) 2014
40 E. Main St., #1156
Newark, DE 19711
www.speedypublishing.co

Ordering Information:
Quantity sales; Special discounts are available on quantity purchases by corporations, associations, and others. For details, contact the "Special Sales Department" at the address above.

-- 1st edition

Manufactured in the United States of America

Table of Contents

Publisher's Notes i

Chapter 1: What Are Green Smoothies? 1

Chapter 2: What Are The Benefits Of Consuming Green Smoothies? . 5

Chapter 3: How To Prepare A Green Smoothie 9

Chapter 4: 10 High Protein Green Smoothie Recipes 16

Chapter 5: 10 Post Workout Green Smoothie Recipes 23

Chapter 6: 10 Smoothie Breakfast Recipes 30

Chapter 7: 10 Green Smoothie Snack Recipes 37

Chapter 8: 10 Green Smoothie Lunch Recipes 45

About the Author 52

More Books by Daisy Williams 54

Publisher's Notes

Disclaimer

This publication is intended to provide helpful and informative material. It is not intended to diagnose, treat, cure, or prevent any health problem or condition, nor is intended to replace the advice of a physician. No action should be taken solely on the contents of this book. Always consult your physician or qualified health-care professional on any matters regarding your health and before adopting any suggestions in this book or drawing inferences from it.

The author and publisher specifically disclaim all responsibility for any liability, loss or risk, personal or otherwise, which is incurred as a consequence, directly or indirectly, from the use or application of any contents of this book.

Any and all product names referenced within this book are the trademarks of their respective owners. None of these owners have sponsored, authorized, endorsed, or approved this book.

Always read all information provided by the manufacturers' product labels before using their products. The author and publisher are not responsible for claims made by manufacturers.

Print Edition 2014

Chapter 1: What Are Green Smoothies?

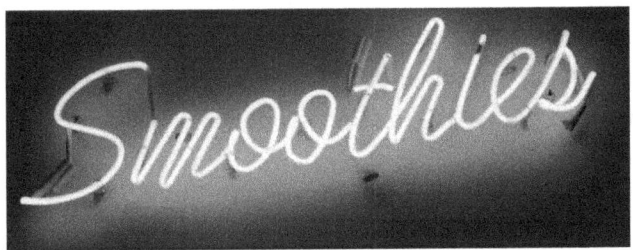

Have you been feeling sluggish, depressed, anxious, irritable, fatigued, or just generally not healthy? If so, then you might want to closely examine your diet, as it's more than likely the culprit behind feeling unwell. Even when we're overworked and stressed out to the max, we should still have the energy to deal with it. Not getting the proper nutrition in your diet is one of the leading causes of the aforementioned health ailments experienced my most people in the world today.

When it comes to eating healthy, smoothies can really add a massive amount of otherwise lacking nutrition to your overall daily diet, especially green smoothies. For those of you who have never had the pleasure of drinking a green smoothie, they're smoothies that contain some element of fresh leafy green vegetables in them, such as kale, spinach, romaine lettuce, mustard greens, parsley, and other delicious green vegetables and herbs.

An example of a green smoothie recipe that many people drink for its nutritional benefits would be a kale spinach banana hemp milk smoothie. Creating it is super easy, as you simply toss the aforementioned ingredients into your blender and puree them into a liquid drink. You can thicken or loosen the green smoothie by adding either more or less almond milk, orange juice, water, or whatever diluter that you decide to add.

A typical green smoothie such as the one that we described above can contain as much as 600% of the daily recommended allowance of vitamin C, vitamin K, vitamin A, calcium, iron, magnesium, potassium, and many other essential vitamins and minerals. You can quite literally take your daily vitamin in the form of a morning breakfast green smoothie, and it will be absorbed by your body much more so than a daily vitamin would be.

When making green smoothies, there are three important tips to consider. First, you should try to use organic locally grown produce only, as it's healthier for you. Second, you should consume your green smoothie with some sort of healthy fat blended into it, such as hemp milk, a little avocado, almond milk, or MCT oil. These healthy fats will dramatically increase your body's absorption of the vast amount of vitamins and minerals contained in the smoothie, as many of them are fat soluble. And thirdly, never add ice cream, sugar, cow's milk, or any other unhealthy ingredients into your green smoothie, as it completely negates the reason for drinking it in the first place.

When making green smoothies, regardless of what you put into them, it's important to have the right tools for the job. In this case you'll need a blender. The higher quality the blender you use, the easier it will be to liquefy the smoothie ingredients. Certain high end blender models on the market today can liquefy a green smoothie in 10 seconds or less. These high powered, sometimes 2 HP machines, generally cost upwards of about $400 per unit.

Another great aspect of green smoothies is that they are super affordable. If you add up the price of a couple handfuls of kale and spinach, plus a banana, some almond milk, and whatever else you add to it, you're more than likely only going to be spending around $4 or less for the whole beverage. That price includes using organic ingredients only. That is an extremely cheap price for a superfood breakfast meal in today's modern world.

When spending money on green smoothie ingredients, or on a high quality blender, you should consider the money spent as an investment in your daily and long term health. Imagine how much more productive you can be if you're eating healthy, which ultimately means you can make more money. Imagine how much money you'll save in medical costs if you're eating really healthy. When you add up the costs of green smoothies, and then factor in all of the benefits that your body will be getting out of them, then it should quickly become clear that its money extremely well spent.

At this point you're probably thinking to yourself, "Green smoothies would probably taste like grass, no thanks". On the contrary! While flavor and taste are completely subjective, if a green smoothie is made properly it can taste far better than a stack of heavy pancakes, or an unhealthy breakfast cereal that's loaded with artificial colors and flavors. When you make green smoothies with bananas, berries, nut milk, and other delicious ingredients, these green smoothies can taste so good that you'll be looking forward to having one all day long. The only time that green smoothies were gross tasting was back in the 80s when no one knew how to make them properly.

Green smoothies are so popular today because they actually have real health benefits, they're not some just crazy diet fad that will come and go. Many peak performance athletes, business titans, tech gurus, and other noteworthy people around the world drink a green smoothie daily, because they can feel what these smoothies are doing to their bodies. They're getting beautiful and radiant skin with clean complexions, regular bowel movements, tons of energy, more mental clarity and focus, more restful sleep, and many other benefits. When your body is getting the nutrition it needs, it will heal itself.

GREEN SMOOTHIES

Ask any doctor and they'll tell you that the root cause of most diseases and illnesses in the human body are caused from tissue inflammation. Many unhealthy foods such as sugar, gluten, dairy, meats, and other common foods that we all eat cause inflammation in the body, which in turn leads to illness. Leafy green vegetables on the other hand, such as those found in green smoothies, are loaded with anti-inflammatory properties, anti-oxidants, and other powerful disease fighting agents.

The best way to get hooked on green smoothies is to start slow. Have one green smoothie every single week. Then bump it up to twice a week. And eventually you'll feel the immediate health benefits from them, and before you know it, you'll be drinking a green smoothie every single day.

Chapter 2: What Are The Benefits Of Consuming Green Smoothies?

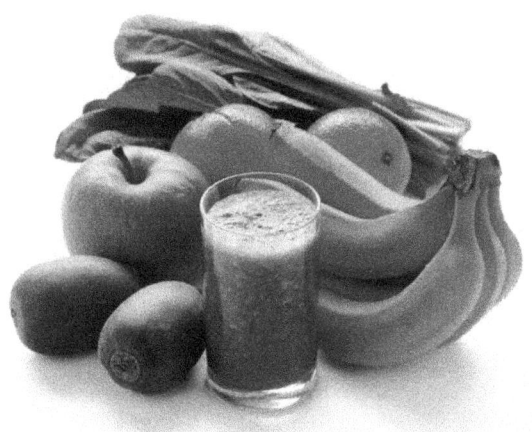

The smoothie craze is not that new. However, green smoothies seem to be creating quite a buzz recently. Health conscious people realize the benefits of eating greens, but many of them find this to be the most unpleasant side of their healthy lifestyles. Consuming green smoothies has rescued the anti-green eaters from their plight.

These drinks are extremely healthy and nutritious. They are mixture of around 60% natural ripe organic fruit, and around 40% pure organic greens. They are a power punch of vital nutrients that the body needs, and they offer a tasty alternative to eating cooked greens.

A green smoothie is a complete food due to the fact it still contains fiber. Fiber is a vital part of the body's elimination system. The smoothies are also very easy for the body to digest. A well-blended smoothie will have greens and fruits in it that now have ruptured cells that can now release the nutrients more readily into the body, and making it easier for them to be assimilated.

Chlorophyll is the life-giving ingredient of greens. Chlorophyll molecules are very similar to human blood molecules in appearance. Even people who are on "raw food" diets don't consume enough greens. You can drink 2 to 3 cups of green smoothies every day, and you will be consuming enough greens to nourish the body, and get all the beneficial nutrients, and they will all be well assimilated.

Because of the sweet flavor of the fruits in these smoothies, children really like them as well. They get a lot of energy and health benefits from green smoothies. Even babies from 6 months and up can benefit from drinking green smoothies. Children are notorious for not wanting to eat their vegetables, but with green smoothies they'll be asking for them.

A green smoothie can be custom-made to suit the taste of the creator. Due to the fruit to veggie ratio favoring the fruits, the taste is dominated by the fruit flavor, making a delicious drink balanced out with healthy greens.

The "juicing" crowd finds their methods to be expensive, time consuming, and messy. That causes many juicers to eventually give up on the whole idea. On the other hand, the smoothie crowd finds green smoothies very easy to create, and quite simple to clean up. You can prepare a green smoothie in under five minutes, clean-up and all.

One thing people don't think about that some have noticed, is that once a person gets used to drinking green smoothies, even if they never liked eating greens their bodies begin to crave them. This is great in the case of children. Even though eating fresh greens is always recommended, a green smoothie will stay fresh in the fridge for as long as 3 days. That means you can take them to work or on trips.

Green smoothies are a great way to lose weight. When your fruit and vegetable intake increases, it gives your body the opportunity to shed off excess fat as well as water build-up by eliminating toxins your body has stored. The great thing about green smoothies and weight is that it can work both ways. Even for those who would like to gain a little, a smoothie can make it easier to drink in some extra calories for putting on weight rather than eating them.

People of all ages can suffer from a lack of mental clarity due to the foods they eat. However, it is more prevalent in older people. Junk foods full of sugar and processed flour, clog up the mind and make the brain feel dull and cloudy. When you drink green smoothies your mind will clear up and you will realize more creativity and clarity of thought. The more you increase your input of healthy foods into your daily diet, and decrease the intake of unhealthy foods, you will see yourself stop craving those junk foods and instead begin to crave the healthy ones.

Green smoothies are quite filling as well. This means less craving for snacks. They also are good for your skin. Many people report a reduction in their acne problems from drinking green smoothies. Women see that the increase in their fluid intake from drinking green smoothies hydrates their skin and actually reduces wrinkles.

Everyone has heard for years how one of the best guards against serious diseases is getting enough vegetables into your diet. Cancer, heart disease, and diabetes are among the serious diseases that fruits and vegetables can help to avoid. The vital nutrients from your smoothie help to boost your immune system. Improving the immune system helps you to resist flu, colds, and viruses that would otherwise take advantage of a weaker immune system.

Some people have problems with digestion. Well, drinking green smoothies can help with that as well. They help you to "detox" and rid your body of unhealthy toxins. It has been proven time and time again, that fruits and vegetables are the key to eliminating bad health problems. Many people before were unable to enjoy such benefits because they were actually repulsed by the taste of greens. But with green smoothies everyone can reap the benefits of greens and enjoy doing it.

It has been recommended by the American Cancer Society, that we eat between five and nine servings per day of fruits and vegetables, for preventing cancer and many other diseases so people who hate the taste of leafy greens, can make a green smoothie that will have a taste that is dominated by mango, pineapple, strawberry, or banana. They never have to taste the carrots, spinach, kale, broccoli, or any other type of vegetables they choose to add.

Getting an excellent dose of antioxidants along with phytonutrients every day, will increase your energy, increase your fiber intake, boost your immune system, clear your mind, and increase your overall quality of life, as you enjoy all the benefits of green smoothies. Grab your blender, open the fridge, and get started today!

Chapter 3: How To Prepare A Green Smoothie

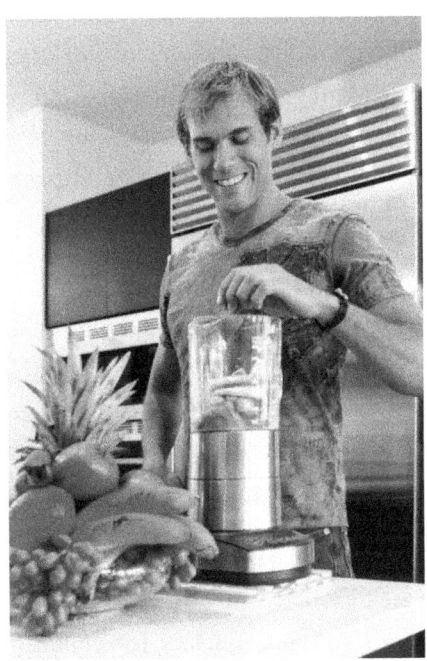

This straightforward recipe is ideal for extremely active individuals who want to sustain a balanced regime, weight management, and prevention of many health related diseases. The fast and simple procedure is well-suited for each person's dynamic lifestyle and is sure to satisfy most consumers. Furthermore, a green smoothie is known to provide enriching gratifications for many users desiring an enhanced nutritional intake.

Regularly consuming a homemade green smoothie is an excellent approach to include fruits and vegetables into one's diet. Vegetables are known to contain the most valuable nutrients, such as essential amino acids, which aid in the building of protein to support muscle mass. In addition, vegetables are plentiful in vitamin A, vitamin C, folate, fiber, and potassium to facilitate the formation of red blood cells, protection against infection, and nourishment of the eyes and skin.

Similarly, this drink is also rich in fresh fruits, counteracting the occasional bitter taste in vegetables. Fruits contain many anti-oxidants, vitamins, minerals, and micronutrients, all of which protect against oxidant stress, disease, and cancers. These compounds also help impede the natural aging of the body such as wrinkling of skin, hair loss, and memory impairments to major illnesses such as AMRD (age-related macular degeneration) of the retina, osteoporosis, colon cancers and Alzheimer's disease.

Along with the drink's valued nutritional content, the convenience of this beverage also appeals to vigorous health advocates. For example, a natural green smoothie can be leisurely consumed in one's home or while one is traveling to work, kids soccer practices, or other scheduled activities. Essentially, the drink's flexibility encourages users to obtain a nutritious supplement regardless of his/her location.

Lastly, this treasured recipe is perfect for children who refuse to consume their daily fruits and vegetables. The blend of sweet and savory ingredients promotes a delicious drink that even kids can truly enjoy. Moreover, this beverage provides youth with energy to successfully participate in stimulating activities and reassures parents that their child is properly developing.

Although fruits and vegetables can eliminate most health problems, many individuals have difficulties incorporating essential nutrients into their daily regime. As such, a simple homemade green smoothie can complement any lifestyle while promoting overall wellness in many individuals. Most importantly, the nutritional effects of this drink will benefit many consumers throughout a lifetime.

Homemade Green Smoothie

Ingredients:
1 large orange, peeled and segmented
½ of a large banana cut into chunks
1¾ cup green grapes
6 large strawberries
¼ Bartlett pear, ripe, seeded, and halved
1 organic apple, cored and chopped
½ avocado, pitted and peeled
2 cups chopped kale
¼ coarsely chopped broccoli
1 cucumber
2 cups spinach, washed
1 large head of organic romaine
½ cup cilantro
½ cup of parsley
5-7 large stalks of chopped organic celery
1 tablespoon flax seed meal (optional)
Pinch of cinnamon or cacao
1/3 cup plain Greek yogurt
¼ cup filtered water
¼ cup milk
1 tablespoon coconut oil
1/3 cup orange juice
½ pineapple juice
Juice of 1 lemon
1 cup ice

Equipment:
Large cutting board
Various assorted bowls
Vegetable/Fruit Peeler
Chef's Knife
High-quality blender

GREEN SMOOTHIES

2 glasses or travel cups
Measuring spoons
Measuring cups
Can opener

Directions:

A green smoothie can be custom-made to suit the taste of the creator. Due to the fruit to veggie ratio favoring the fruits, the taste is dominated by the fruit flavor, making a delicious drink balanced out with healthy greens.

The "juicing" crowd finds their methods to be expensive, time consuming, and messy. That causes many juicers to eventually give up on the whole idea. On the other hand, the smoothie crowd finds green smoothies very easy to create, and quite simple to clean up. You can prepare a green smoothie in under five minutes, clean-up and all.

Pour filtered water, milk, coconut oil, pineapple, orange, and lemon juice into a high-quality blender.

1. Next, add all chopped vegetables including avocado, kale, broccoli, cucumber, spinach, romaine lettuce, cilantro, parsley, and celery.
2. Secure lid and puree on low speed for 35-40 seconds or until the mixture exhibits a thick consistency.
3. Gradually increase the speed and include the sliced fruits: oranges, banana, grapes, strawberries, pears, and apples.
4. While maintaining a medium speed, add remaining ingredients, ice and yogurt.
5. Lastly, slowly combine flax seed meal and cinnamon.
6. Continue blending and adding water until creamy or until the desired thickness is obtained.
7. After effectively blending all the ingredients, taste the concoction and adjust the mixture as necessary.

8. Pour the beverage into glasses or travel cups and enjoy an effortless nutritious drink.

Green Smoothie Possible Add-Ins

With practice, individuals will perfect this standard green smoothie recipe and gradually begin to create a healthy beverage which more accurately corresponds to their taste buds. Moreover, consumers should recognize the many variations of a nutritious green smoothie and are encouraged to experiment with the following additional ingredients:

<u>**Fruits:**</u>
Peach
Cherries
Nectarine
Mango
Pineapple
Honeydew melon,
Blueberries
Blackberries
Golgi berries
Raspberries
Pink grapefruit
Young coconut meat
Unsweetened shredded coconut

<u>**Vegetables:**</u>
Carrots
Collard green leaves
Ginger, hemp seeds
Chia seeds

<u>**Liquids:**</u>
Vanilla
Coconut water

Coconut milk
Nut milks

Miscellaneous:
Protein powders
Blackstrap molasses
Spirulina
Bee pollen
Lacuma
Cocoa nibs
Raw gluten free oats
Sprouted buckwheat groats
Matcha tea powder
Cayenne
Chlorella
Honey

Tips:

In order to create the best green smoothie, some additional considerations should be acknowledged.

- Utilizing a powerful blender will ensure the fruits and vegetables are pureed properly. Before creating the drink, ensure that the blender will effectively crush the oranges, spinach, ice, etc.
- When storing this nutritious drink, pour in an air-tight container and freeze. Also, remember to remove from the freezer about thirty minutes before consumption to encourage efficient thawing practices. In addition, this drink can also be stored in the refrigerator.
- However, for optimal nutrient content, the smoothie should be immediately consumed while the ingredients are fresh. Similarly, users are also encouraged to limit food

consumption 40 minutes before and after drinking the beverage.
- Simply thicken the mixture by adding ice if too much liquid is accidently added. In contrast, liquefy the drink by including more water.
- Most importantly, when preparing this recipe, start the blender on the slowest speed and gradually increase to higher speeds to effectively crush the bigger ingredients.

This drink is perfect for the entire family. Enjoy a green smoothie and truly experience the fun in consuming fruits and vegetables.

CHAPTER 4: 10 HIGH PROTEIN GREEN SMOOTHIE RECIPES

Here are 10 green smoothie recipes that are not only delicious but nutritious, easily digestible, high in fiber, and helps you consume your 5 a days that are important to consume on a daily basis. They will give you energy and keep your body regular.

FIGGY GREEN MONSTER SMOOTHIE

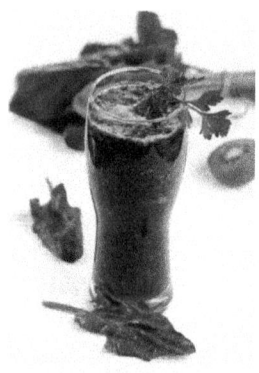

Ingredients:
1½ -2 cups lightly packed spinach
1 banana (frozen bananas will make the smoothie thicker but non frozen will work just as well)
4 four figs (with stems removed and halved)
1 cup of milk
2 ice cubes

Directions:
1. Blend all ingredients until combined and serve.

PEANUT BUTTER COCOA SPINACH GREEN SMOOTHIE

Ingredients:
1 frozen banana
2-3 handfuls of spinach
2 tsp. peanut butter (creamy not crunchy)
2 tsp. cocoa powder
1–1½ cups of soy milk

Directions:
1. Blend together a frozen banana, two or three handfuls of spinach, two table spoons of peanut butter creamy not crunchy, two table spoons of cocoa powder, and one or one and a half cups of soy milk.
2. You can also use regular or almond milk which ever you prefer to use.

LEMONY GREEN SMOOTHIE WITH SORREL AND STRAWBERRIES

Ingredients:
2 big handfuls of sorrel stems and leaves
Juice of one lemon
1½ avocado flesh (not the inside of the avocado just the outer rind)
3 red strawberries
Ice
Water

Directions:
1. Combine two big handfuls of sorrel stems and leaves, the juice of one lemon, one half of an avocado flesh, 3 strawberries, a handful of ice, and a splash of water.
2. Pour and enjoy this yummy smoothie.

GREEN SMOOTHIES

RED GRAPE SMOOTHIE

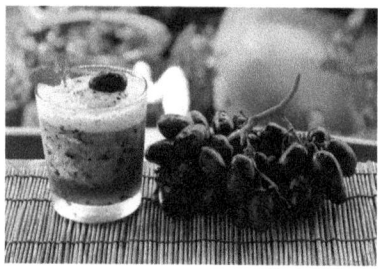

Ingredients:
2 cups of red seedless grapes
1 cup of greens (kale lettuce or spinach)
1 chopped medium pear (remove core)
½ cup frozen pumpkin puree
¾ cup coconut water
Ice

Directions:
1. Blend two cups of red seedless grapes, one cup of greens kale lettuce or spinach, one medium pear that is cored and chopped up, one half cup frozen pumpkin puree, 3/4 cup coconut water, and some ice.
2. Another refreshing green smoothie to be enjoyed by all.

CARROT CAKE GREEN MONSTER SMOOTHIE

Ingredients:
2 small or 1 large carrot with greens or spinach
1 ripe banana
½ cup of skin milk
½ cup of water
⅛ cup of oats
1 tbsp. hemp powder (optional)
½ tsp. cinnamon
4-5 ice cubes

Directions:
1. Blend all ingredients until combined and serve.

FESTIVE ROMAINE AND APPLE GREEN SMOOTHIE WITH CINNAMON

This is a great smoothie for the holidays with the cinnamon and because of the different ingredients you hardly taste the romaine lettuce.

Ingredients:
½-1 bunch of fresh romaine lettuce (chopped up roughly)
1-2 apples (chopped up)
1 banana (chopped up)
½ tsp. ground cinnamon
1 cup of water
1 cup of ice

Directions:
1. Blend all ingredients together and enjoy!

TROPICAL VITAMIN C BLAST GREEN MONSTER SMOOTHIE

Ingredients:
1½ loosely packed cups of spinach
3 leaves of fresh parsley
1 frozen banana
5 small pieces of frozen mango
Handful frozen pineapple
¼ cup orange juice
Soy milk (or other milk)
Sweetener

Directions:
1. Blend all of the ingredients except for sweetener together in a blender.
2. Add sweetener to taste.

GREEN MACHINE SMOOTHIE

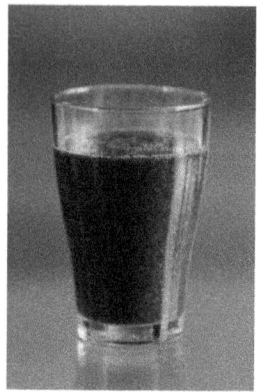

Ingredients:
1 chopped granny smith apple (or pear)
2 cups of kale
1 lime or lemon
½ cup of orange juice
2 tsp. of ginger
1/3 cup of a chopped frozen banana

Directions:
1. Blend all ingredients until combined and serve.

GREEN AFTER WORKOUT SMOOTHIE

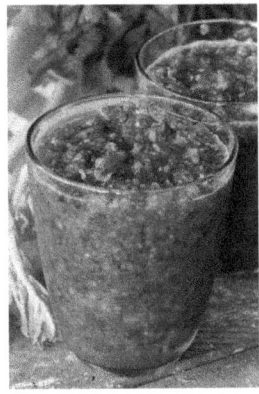

Ingredients:
10 ounces of water
½ scoop of your favorite protein powder
½ cup of Greek yogurt
1 handful of spinach
1 tsp. ground fresh flaxseed
½ tsp xanthium gum (thickening agent)
3 ice cubes

Directions:
1. Blend all ingredients until combined and serve.

WHITE PEACH, ORANGE AND ROMAINE LETTUCE SMOOTHIE

This is a very simple recipe with only a few ingredients but tastes so good.

Ingredients:
1 white peach (pitted and chopped)
2 oranges (peeled and chopped)
4-6 romaine lettuce leaves
1 cup of ice

Directions:

1. Use a blender to combine all the ingredients and serve.

All ten of these green smoothies have a few things in common; they all will help boost your energy. They are all very high in fiber because so they help regulate your body and keep your system clean.

CHAPTER 5: 10 POST WORKOUT GREEN SMOOTHIE RECIPES

After an intense workout, a green smoothie is just the thing to replenish fluids, and help reinforce the results you want from your exercise commitment to good health. Here are 10 recipes for tasty green smoothies that will give you the nutrients your body needs. With these 10 diverse recipes, anybody should be able to find a recipe they enjoy.

BASIC SMOOTHIE

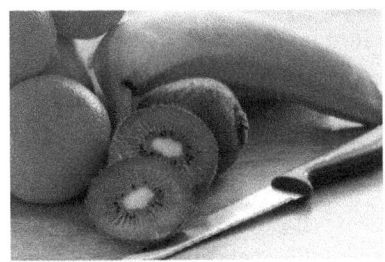

Ingredients:

2 peeled oranges
1 banana
1 kiwi
1 cup of spinach
Water

Directions:

This smoothie is a standard fixture among green smoothie enthusiasts. It is easy to make for beginners and very popular.
1. Take two peeled oranges and remove the seeds before adding them to the blender.
2. Next add one banana and one kiwi.

GREEN SMOOTHIES

3. Take a cup of spinach and add it to the mix.
4. Pour a cup of water over it all.
5. Mix well until the mixture is smooth enough to drink like a milkshake.

ORANGE JUICE SMOOTHIE

Ingredients:
1 cup of orange
1 orange (halved)
1 green kiwi (halved)
1 bunch of spinach
¼ head of lettuce

Directions:
1. Peel the orange before adding it into the blender.
2. Spoon out the kiwi into the blender.
3. Mix all the ingredients together until the drink is creamy and enjoy the tangy taste.

EASY DIGESTION SMOOTHIE

For when your stomach may be complaining, this smoothie is even easier to drink and digest than the normally easy-to-digest green smoothie usually is.

Ingredients:
1¾ cups of water
1 one kiwi
3 mandarin oranges
1 banana
1 stalk of rape leaves (one stalk, not a bunch)

*If you substitute the recipe for regular oranges, you will only need half as much, due to the larger size of typical oranges.

Directions:
1. Blend everything together until you reach the desired level of smoothness.

*The consistency of this drink should be a little thinner than a typical green smoothie.

LIMEADE SMOOTHIE

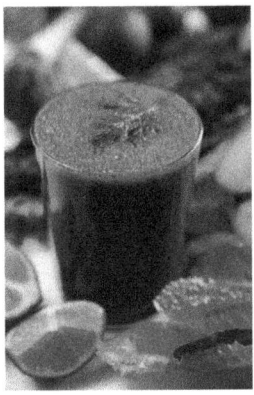

Ingredients:
1 cup of coconut water
1 cup of either milk or water

Vegetables
½ cup of cilantro
1½ cup kale
1 lime (peeled)
2-3 bananas
1 inch of ginger

Directions:
1. Add the liquids, cilantro and kale together into a blender and blend until they are smooth.
2. Add the other ingredients and keep blending until the smoothie reaches the same consistency.

ASIAN SMOOTHIE

Ingredients:
⅓ pack of grape
1 sliced apple
2 sliced pears
¼ tsp. cinnamon
2 cups water

Directions:
1. Mix the ingredients together for a smoothie that can fill a one liter bottle.

An alternative recipe uses half a pineapple, half of one yellow paprika and a whole grapefruit.

PEACH AND LETTUCE SMOOTHIE

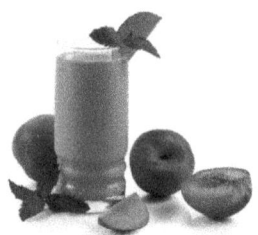

Ingredients:
4 peaches
1 cup of lettuce (or baby leaf)
½ slice of lemon
1 banana
1 cup of water

Directions:
1. The peaches can be blended without peeling them, but make sure to remove the seeds.

2. For the lettuce or baby leaf, make sure to use the darkest and greenest parts for the best results.
3. Mix every ingredient at once until nice and smooth.

SUMMER SMOOTHIE

For a smoothie with a tinge of summer in it, why not use watermelon?

Ingredients:
1 orange
½ an apple
1 frozen banana
Watermelon
1½ cups water
3-4 rape leaves (large)

Directions:
1. Cut all the fruits into small slices.
2. Prepare the watermelon with anywhere from five to seven pieces of roughly one-inch slices, depending on how strongly you want to enjoy the watermelon taste.
3. Add one-and-a-half cups of water, and mix together until smooth.
4. Next add three to four large rape leaves into the blender and mix until you get a light green, smooth drink with a taste of summer.

SOY SMOOTHIE

Ingredients:
1 cup of the healthy lactose-free alternative
1 golden kiwi instead
1 apple
1 frozen banana
30-50 grams of baby leaf

GREEN SMOOTHIES

Directions:
1. Cut the kiwi in half and cut the apple into small slices
2. Add all the ingredients to your blender and after a minute or two, it should be smooth.

AVOCADO SMOOTHIE

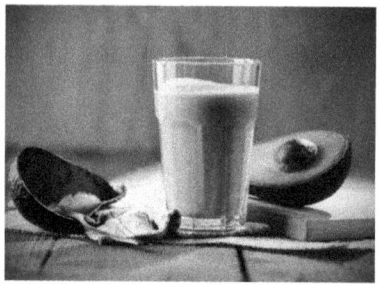

Ingredients:
1 cup of water
1 avocado
2 tomatoes
2 bananas
3-4 tablespoons of honey
2 tablespoons of lemon juice

Directions:
1. Cut all the vegetables and fruits into small chunks and then add them to the blender.
2. Next, put in the tablespoons of honey and lemon juice.
3. Last, add the water.
4. Blend it all together and keep in mind that if you want a thicker smoothie, you can keep the water down to half a cup.

AUTUMN HARVEST SMOOTHIE

This smoothie uses many ingredients that are freshest in autumn.

Ingredients:
1 cup turnip greens

2 Asian pears
½ Lemons (seeds removed)
Figs

<u>Directions:</u>
1. Blend together with a cup of water for a great autumn smoothie.

CHAPTER 6: 10 SMOOTHIE BREAKFAST RECIPES

SUPER GREEN SMOOTHIE RECIPE

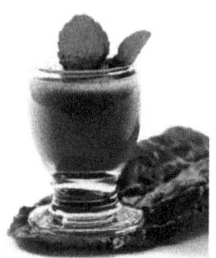

Ingredients:
1 handful of fresh kale
1 handful of fresh spinach
1 handful of fresh Swiss chard
1 large peeled banana
2 tsp. of fresh squeezed lime juice
2 cups of vanilla almond milk
½ cup of crushed ice

Directions:
1. Rinse all of your green under cold running water.
2. Remove the thick stalks and stems from the greens.
3. Add all of the ingredients into your blender.
4. Puree them until they're fully liquefied.
5. Serve the smoothie immediately while it's cold.

KALE SPINACH BANANA HEMP MILK SMOOTHIE RECIPE

Ingredients:
1 large handful of fresh kale
1 large handful of fresh spinach

1 large peeled banana
2 cups of hemp milk

Directions:
1. Thoroughly rinse your produce under cold running tap water.
2. Discard the tough kale stalk and thick spinach stems.
3. Place all of the ingredients into your blender.
4. Puree the ingredients for approximately 20 to 40 seconds, or until the ingredients are completely liquefied.
5. Serve the smoothie immediately.

DELICIOUS PROTEIN SMOOTHIE RECIPE

Ingredients:
1 scoop of pea protein powder
2 large peeled bananas
½ cup of crushed ice
1/8 cup of raw unsalted almonds
1/8 cup of raw rolled oats
2 cups of fresh squeezed orange juice

Directions:
1. Freshly squeeze two cups of orange juice.
2. The orange juice can have pulp or be pulp free - your choice.
3. Add ingredients and blend until ingredients are liquefied.
4. Serve immediately.

GREEN SMOOTHIES

SPINACH BANANA STRAWBERRY PROTEIN SMOOTHIE RECIPE

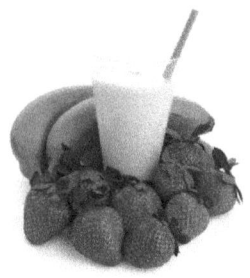

Ingredients:
1 large handful of fresh spinach
1 large peeled banana
½ cup of fresh stemless-strawberries
2 cups of almond milk
2 tbsp. of hemp protein powder
½ cup of crushed ice
2 tbsp. of fresh squeezed lemon juice

Directions:
1. Rinse your kale and strawberries under cool running water.
2. Discard the tough kale stalk and strawberry stems / greens.
3. Add all of these delicious ingredients into your blender container.
4. Serve immediately.

CREAMY BANANA WALNUT DATE SMOOTHIE RECIPE

Ingredients:
3 medium size pitted dates
2 large peeled bananas
1/8 cup of shelled unsalted walnuts
1 cup of unsweetened almond milk
1 cup of freshly squeezed orange juice
½ Cup of Crushed Ice

Directions:
1. Remove the pits from your dates.
2. Remove any shell pieces from your walnuts.
3. Freshly squeeze one cup of orange juice.
4. Add all of the ingredients into your blender.
5. Puree until totally smooth.
6. Serve the smoothie immediately.

CREAMY WATERMELON ORANGE SMOOTHIE RECIPE

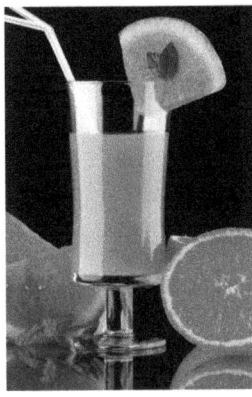

Ingredients:

2 cups of fresh cubed seedless watermelon

1 cup of unsweetened rice milk

1 cup of fresh squeezed orange juice

1 dash of fresh ground cloves

½ cup of crushed ice

Directions:
1. Prepare your cubed watermelon.
2. Make sure to remove all of the watermelon seeds, as blending even one will ruin your smoothie.
3. Freshly squeeze one cup of orange juice.
4. Add all of these sweet and delicious ingredients into your blender.
5. Puree until smooth. Serve immediately while cold.

GREEN SMOOTHIES

SIMPLE PROTEIN SMOOTHIE RECIPE

Ingredients:
2 large peeled bananas
1 scoop of hemp protein powder
2 cups of premade orange juice
½ cup of crushed ice

Directions:
1. Add ingredients into your blender container.
2. Blend on high speed until the smoothie becomes totally liquefied.
3. To thicken the smoothie, add more ice.
4. To loosen it add more orange juice.
5. Serve the smoothie immediately in a tall drink glass.
6. Feel free to garnish the smoothie with a dash of fresh ground cinnamon.

DAISY'S FAMOUS APPLE BANANA YOGURT SMOOTHIE RECIPE

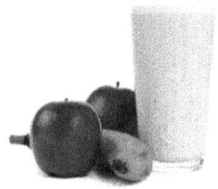

Ingredients:
1/8 cup of raw rolled oats
4 fresh skinless apple slices
1 large peeled banana
1 dash of ground ginger
1 dash of ground cinnamon
1 cup of peach yogurt
8 raw unsalted almonds
1 cup of premade apple juice

1 cup of cold water

½ cup of crushed ice

Directions:

1. Add all of these ingredients into your blender container.
2. Blend the ingredients for 40 seconds or until the smoothie is totally liquefied.
3. Serve immediately.

ANTIOXIDANT SUPERFOOD SMOOTHIE RECIPE

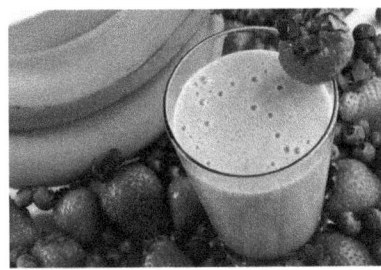

Ingredients:

½ cup of Fresh Blueberries

½ cup of Fresh Strawberries

2 tbsp. of Acai Powder

½ cup of Crushed Ice

1 peeled Banana

2 cups of Fresh Squeezed Orange Juice

Directions:

1. Thoroughly rinse your fresh berries under cool running water.
2. Remove the berry stems.
3. Freshly squeeze two cups of orange juice.
4. Place all of these super food ingredients into a blender.
5. Blend until the smoothie is totally liquefied.
6. Serve immediately.

CARROT PINEAPPLE BANANA SMOOTHIE RECIPE

Ingredients:
¼ cup of peeled chopped carrots
¼ cup of fresh pineapple chunks
2 large peeled bananas
2 cups of unsweetened almond milk
1 cup of crushed ice
1 tsp. of liquid vanilla extract

Directions:
1. Rinse your produce under running water.
2. Peel your carrots.
3. Add ingredients into your blender container.
4. Blend until the smoothie is totally consistent and even.
5. Serve immediately in a tall drink glass.
6. Garnish with a dash of fresh ground cloves.

Chapter 7: 10 Green Smoothie Snack Recipes

This is a list of smoothies that can be made to drink as a snack. The taste of smoothies can vary from person to person because of individual likes and dislikes, but all of these smoothies can be adjusted to accommodate anyone's taste buds. Just add a little more of this or less of that. Or just add a tablespoon of a natural sweetener. But in each recipe the flavors are a refreshing mix of ingredients.

The old fashioned oats are added in some recipes to give more body to the smoothie and adding more fiber to the human body will keep you satisfied between meals. The oats and water can be mixed beforehand in a container, if it is too time consuming to do it when the smoothie is being prepared.

There is great flavor and nutrients in the stem of the mint sprig. So don't just use the leaves, add the whole sprig.

STRAWBERRY CARROT SMOOTHIE

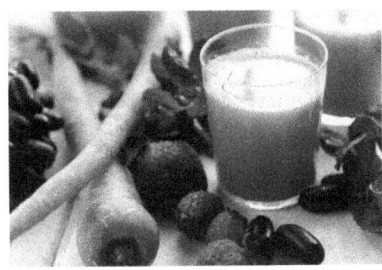

Ingredients:
½ cup water
¼ old fashioned rolled oats

GREEN SMOOTHIES

½ cup apple juice
½ cup strawberries frozen
1 carrot washed and chopped into chunks
1 cup spinach

Directions:
1. In a blender combine water and oats.
2. Let it stand for 15 minutes.
3. Then add the apple juice, strawberries, carrots, and spinach.
4. Start blending on low to break up the big pieces, and then blend on high until the desired consistency is reached.
5. Water can be added to thin the smoothie if it is too thick.

BANANA BEET SMOOTHIE

Ingredients:
½ cup coconut milk
1 frozen banana
1 small beet peeled and cut into chunks or half of a large beet
1 cup spinach
¼ cup raw cashews

Directions:
1. In a blender combine coconut milk, banana, beet, spinach, and cashews.
2. Blend on low to break up the pieces, and then increase the speed to high.
3. Blend until the desired consistency is reached.
4. Water can be added to thin the smoothie if it is too thick.

BLUEBERRY BANANA SMOOTHIE

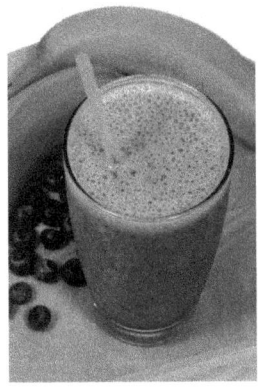

Ingredients:
½ cup coconut milk
1 cup spinach
½ cup frozen blueberries
1 celery stalk cut into chunks
½ frozen banana

Directions:
1. In a blender combine coconut milk, spinach, blueberries, celery and banana
2. Blend on low to break up the pieces, and then increase the speed to high.
3. Blend until the desired consistency is reached.
4. Water can be added to thin the smoothie if it is too thick.

APPLE CARROT SMOOTHIE

Ingredients:
½ cup water
¼ cup old fashioned oats
1 apple (cored and cut into chunks)
1 carrot (cut into chunks)
1 cup kale

½ cup raisins
3 ice cubes
1 tbsp. flax seed
½ tsp. cinnamon
1 tbsp. lemon juice

Directions:
1. In a blender combine water and oats.
2. Let stand for 15 minutes.
3. Add apple, carrot, kale, raisins, ice cubes, flax seed, cinnamon, and lemon juice.
4. Blend on low to break up the chunks, and then increase the speed to high.
5. Blend until the desired consistency is reached.
6. Add more water to thin the smoothie if it is too thick.

APPLE CELERY SMOOTHIE

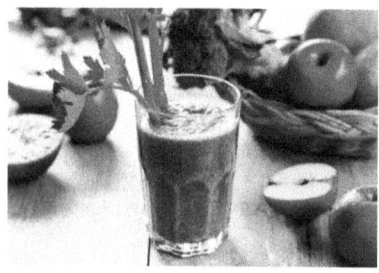

Ingredients:
½ cup tomato juice
1 celery stalk chopped into chunks
1 cup collard greens
1 apple (cored and cut into chunks)
1 tbsp. of Tabasco sauce
3 ice cubes

Directions:
1. In a blender mix tomato juice, celery, collards, apple, Tabasco sauce, and ice.
2. Blend on low to break up the chunks, then increase speed to high.
3. Blend until the desired consistency is reached.
4. Water can be added to thin the smoothie if it is too thick.

CUCUMBER MINT SMOOTHIE

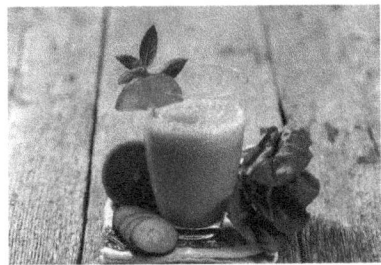

Ingredients:
½ cup water
¼ cup old fashioned rolled oats
½ cup apple juice
½ a cucumber (cut into chunks)
1 cup spinach
1 mint sprig (the whole sprig)
3 ice cubes
1 tbsp. lime juice

Directions:
1. In a blender combine water and oats.
2. Let stand for 15 minutes.
3. Add apple juice, cucumber, spinach, mint, ice, and lime juice to the blender.
4. Blend on low to break up the pieces, and then increase the speed to high.
5. Blend until the desired consistency is reached.

GREEN SMOOTHIES

6. If the smoothie is too thick, then use water to thin.

ALMOND BANANA SMOOTHIE

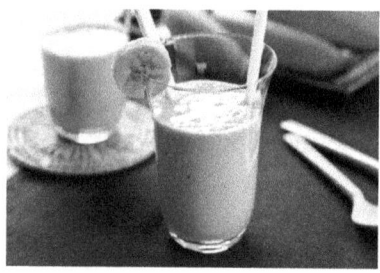

Ingredients:
½ cup water
¼ cup old fashioned rolled oats
½ cup almond milk
½ a banana (frozen)
1 cup Swiss Chard
1 celery stalk cut into chunks
½ cup cranberries frozen

Directions:
1. In a blender combine water and oats.
2. Let stand for 15 minutes.
3. Next, add almond milk, banana, chard, celery, and cranberries.
4. Blend until the desired consistency is reached.
5. Water can be added if smoothie is too thick.

BLUEBERRY CARROT SMOOTHIE

Ingredients:
½ cup coconut milk
½ cup blueberries frozen
1 carrot cut into chunks
1 cup spinach
3 basil leaves
1 tbsp. honey

1 tbsp. lemon juice

Directions:
1. In a blender combine coconut milk, blueberries, carrot, spinach, basil, honey, and lemon juice.
2. Blend on low to break up the pieces, then increase the speed to high.
3. Blend until the desired consistency is reached.
4. Add water is the smoothie is too thick.

RASPBERRY BANANA SMOOTHIE

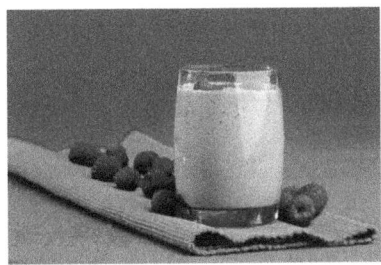

Ingredients:
½ cup water
¼ cup old fashioned rolled oats
½ cup almond milk
½ cup raspberries (frozen)
½ a banana (frozen)
1 cup spinach
½ cup almonds

Directions:
1. In a blender combine water and oats.
2. Let stand for 15 minutes.
3. Next, add almond milk, raspberries, banana, spinach, and almonds.
4. Blend on low to break up the pieces, and then increase the speed to high.
5. Blend until the desired consistency is reached.

6. Add water if the smoothie is too thick.

STRAWBERRY CUCUMBER SMOOTHIE

Ingredients:
½ cup orange juice
½ cup strawberries (frozen)
½ a cucumber
1 cup kale
1 sprig of mint leaves (use the whole sprig)

Directions:
1. In a blender combine orange juice, strawberries, cucumber, kale, and mint.
2. Blend on low to break up the pieces, and then increase the speed to high.
3. Blend until the desired consistency is reached.
4. Water can be added if the smoothie is too thick.

Chapter 8: 10 Green Smoothie Lunch Recipes

KALE SWISS CHARD PARSLEY GREEN SMOOTHIE

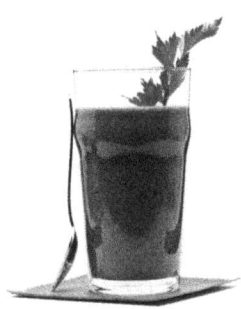

Ingredients:
1 handful of fresh kale
1 handful of fresh Swiss chard
1 very small handful of fresh parsley
½ cup of crushed ice
2 cups of vanilla rice milk
1 large peeled banana
1 dash of ground ginger

Directions:
1. Rinse your greens under cold tap water.
2. Remove any tough stems or stalks from the greens.
3. Add all of these ingredients into a blender.
4. Puree until the smoothie reaches a desired consistency.
5. Serve immediately while the smoothie is cold.

GREEN SMOOTHIES

SPINACH KALE COLLARD GREENS BANANA SMOOTHIE

Ingredients:
1 handful of fresh baby spinach
1 handful of fresh baby leaf kale
1 handful of fresh collard greens
1 large peeled banana
1 cup of vanilla yogurt
½ cup of crushed ice
1 dash of fresh ground ginger
2 cups of fresh squeezed orange juice

Directions:
1. Thoroughly rinse all of your fresh delicious greens under cold running water. Remove any stems, stalks, or hard fibrous parts from then add 2 freshly squeezed cups of orange juice.
2. Blend all of these ingredients together until a creamy green smoothie forms. Serve immediately cold.

BEET GREENS SPINACH BLUEBERRY SMOOTHIE

Ingredients:
1 handful of fresh baby spinach
1 handful of fresh beet greens
½ cup of fresh blueberries (remove stems)
2 cups of sweetened almond milk
1 large peeled banana
1 cup of low fat vanilla yogurt

Directions:
1. Remove the stalk and stems from your veggies and berries.
2. Wash them under cool water.
3. Combine ingredients into your blender container.
4. Blend at high speed until liquefied.
5. Serve smoothie in a tall highball drink glass.

DANDELION GREENS KALE BANANA SMOOTHIE

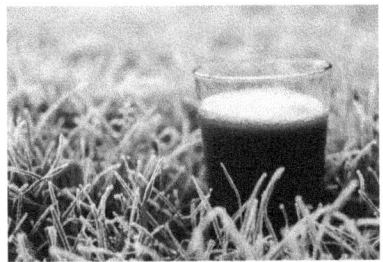

Ingredients:
1 handful of fresh kale
1 handful of fresh dandelion greens
2 large peeled bananas
2 cups of unsweetened hemp milk

Directions:
1. Wash and rinse your greens under cold water.
2. Remove stems or stalks from the veggies.
3. Combine ingredients into your blender.
4. Puree them until smooth.
5. Serve immediately.

BOK CHOY SPINACH BANANA SMOOTHIE

Ingredients:
1 handful of fresh bok choy
1 handful of fresh baby leaf spinach
2 large peeled bananas
2 cups of unsweetened hemp milk
2 tbsp. of freshly squeezed lemon juice

Directions:
1. Wash and rinse greens under cool water.
2. Remove any tough thick stems and stalks.
3. Combine ingredients into your blender container.
4. Puree until the smoothie is fully liquefied.

5. Serve the cold smoothie in a tall drink glass.

SPINACH TURNIP GREENS STRAWBERRY SMOOTHIE

Ingredients:
1 handful of fresh turnip greens
1 handful of baby leaf spinach
½ cup of fresh strawberries (remove stems)
1 large peeled banana
1 cup of almond yogurt
½ cup of ice
2 cups of premade orange juice

Directions:
1. Clean greens and strawberries under cold water.
2. Discard any stems or stalks from the produce.
3. Blend all of these ingredients at high speed for 40 seconds, or until the smoothie is creamy and consistent.
4. Serve immediately in a tall smoothie glass.

PINEAPPLE KALE PEACH BANANA SMOOTHIE

Ingredients:
3 large handfuls of fresh baby leaf kale
2 large peeled bananas
½ cup of fresh cubed pineapple
½ cup of fresh cubed peach
½ cup of crushed ice
2 cups of coconut water
1 dash of freshly ground cloves

Directions:
1. Clean produce under running water.
2. Discard the tough kale stalk.
3. Place all of these ingredients into your blender and puree them on high speed.

4. Serve immediately.

KALE POWDER SUPER PROTEIN SMOOTHIE

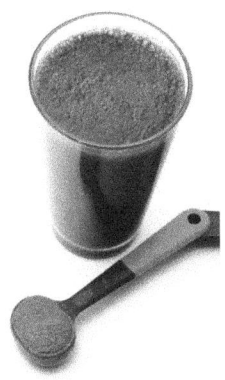

Ingredients:
1/8 cup of organic kale powder
2 large peeled bananas
1 scoop of hemp protein powder
2 cups of unsweetened hemp milk
½ cup of crushed ice
2 tbsp. of fresh squeezed lime juice

Directions:
1. Combine ingredients into your blender container.
2. Puree on high speed until the smoothie is even and consistent.
3. Serve the smoothie immediately in a tall highball drink glass.

SPINACH MANGO BANANA SMOOTHIE

Ingredients:
3 handfuls of fresh spinach
1 large peeled banana
1 cup of fresh ripe mango
½ cup of crushed ice
2 cups of premade orange juice
1 dash of fresh ground nutmeg

Directions:
1. Clean produce under cold running tap water.
2. Remove stems from the spinach.
3. Combine ingredients into your blender.
4. Puree until totally smooth.
5. Serve the ice cold smoothie immediately in a tall highball drink glass.

SPINACH KALE MUSTARD GREENS SMOOTHIE

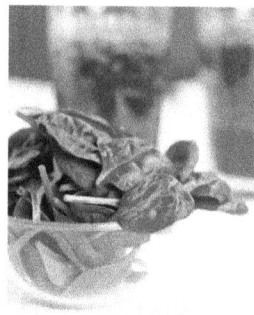

Ingredients:
1 handful of fresh spinach
1 handful of fresh kale
1 tiny handful of fresh mustard greens
1 large fresh banana
½ cup of fresh papaya
½ cup of crushed ice
2 cups of unsweetened rice milk

Directions:
1. Wash and rinse all of your produce under cool tap water.
2. Discard any stems or fibrous stalk from the greens.
3. Place all of these ingredients in your blender container.
4. Blend on high speed until the smoothie reaches a desired consistency.

5. Serve the smoothie in a tall glass.

ABOUT THE AUTHOR

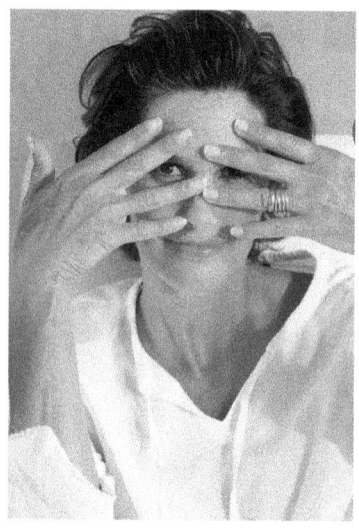

Author and chef Daisy Williams is passionate about clean and healthy eating, but she knows that it can seem next to impossible to someone just embarking on a food journey. It took years for her to move from the all-American diet processed and chemical-ridden convenience food to a healthier lifestyle that draws true nourishment from organic, whole foods. Now that she's made the transition herself, she loves helping people realize that there is a healthier way and that it's not as hard as you might think!

Eating clean didn't come easily to Daisy—her food journey started out of pure necessity. After being constantly ill for years and trying just about every medicine under the sun, she finally tried the nutrition angle as a last-ditch effort. A friend had advised reducing the chemicals in her diet, and since nothing else seemed to be working, she figured there was nothing to lose. Within weeks it became clear that nutrition was a huge factor impacting her health concerns! And thus her passion for clean eating was born.

Daisy is convinced that most people can improve their quality of life by adjusting their nutritional lifestyle. And she wants people considering clean eating to know that it's not impossible; in fact, it's delicious! Her books feature some fantastic recipes, from clean eating and green smoothie recipes that you'll love. Her dream is that through her story, people will be inspired to make healthy changes even before their health is suffering.

More Books by Daisy Williams

Clean Eating: Your Guide to Eating Clean

Clean Eating Recipes: Jumpstart Weight Loss with 70 Clean Eating Recipes

Paleo Slow Cooker Recipes: The Best Paleo Diet Recipes for Your Slow Cooker

www.ingramcontent.com/pod-product-compliance
Ingram Content Group UK Ltd.
Pitfield, Milton Keynes, MK11 3LW, UK
UKHW022120230426
12048UKWH00010BA/621